# EVERYTHING ABOUT

# BODY TYPE DIET

Complete Nutritional Cookbook, Foods, Meal Plan, Recipes To Understand Your Somatotype Crafting Your Ideal Diet And Building A Healthier You

# DR. ALVIN BRANTLEY

© 2023 ALVIN BRANTLEY

All rights reserved. No part of this book may be reproduced, stored, or transmitted in any form or by any means, electronic, mechanical, photocopying, recording, scanning, or otherwise, without the prior written permission of the author.

## Disclaimer

The information provided in this book is intended for general informational purposes only. It is not a substitute for professional medical advice, diagnosis, or treatment.

You should not use the information in this book for diagnosing or treating a health problem or disease by self decision. Always seek the advice of your physician or other qualified health provider with any questions you may have regarding a medical condition.

The author and publisher of this book make no representations or warranties with respect to the accuracy, applicability, fitness, or completeness of the contents of this book. The information contained in this book is based on the author's research and experience, and it is shared with the understanding that the author is not engaged in rendering medical, health, or any other kind of professional advice for you by this book.

The author does not endorse or promote any specific products, brands, or companies related to the contents provided in this book.

Any mention of products or services in this book is for informational purposes only and does not constitute an endorsement.

The author has not entered into any affiliate marketing agreements and has not signed any endorsement deals with individuals, organizations, or companies.

Readers are encouraged to consult with their healthcare providers before making any dietary or lifestyle chaSnges based on the information provided in this book. The author and publisher disclaim any liability for the decisions made by readers based on the information in this book.

# Contents

# Introduction

For everyone aiming to maximize their fitness and health, it is essential to understand the fundamentals of body types. Everybody's body is different, and classifying these variations can give important information about the best diet and exercise regimens. The foundation of the body types concept is the notion that individuals can be categorized into unique groups, each with unique traits. Understanding these body kinds better would enable people to modify their lifestyles to better suit their physiological requirements.

Identifying Body Forms

Three main categories are identified to classify body types: ectomorph, mesomorph, and endomorph. These divisions are predicated on a confluence of elements like body composition, metabolism, and bone structure. It is crucial to comprehend the characteristics that set each body type apart to develop individualized plans for general well-being, fitness, and health. Every body type has advantages and disadvantages of its own, thus it's critical for people to accept and value their individual qualities.

The Meaning of Ectomorph, Mesomorph, and Endomorph

Ectomorphs are defined by their slim, lean bodies, which frequently have long limbs and a quick metabolism. It could be difficult for these people to put on weight and muscular mass. Conversely, mesomorphs typically have a more athletic and muscular frame. Their metabolism is in between that of ectomorphs and endomorphs, hence they typically have an easier time gaining and maintaining muscle. Endomorphs tend to be softer and rounder in form, and they are more likely to accumulate body fat. Comprehending these disparities is crucial in customizing exercise and dietary regimens to meet the unique requirements of every body type.

Finding Your Ideal Body Type

Finding your body type is a crucial first step in customizing your workout and wellness regimen. Many techniques, including evaluating physical attributes, examining metabolism, and taking into account the body's reaction to exercise, can assist people in identifying their predominant body type.

It is important to understand that a lot of people can have a mix of various body types, with one dominating the others. Equipped with this understanding, people can make well-informed choices regarding their food, exercise regimen, and general way of living to attain the best outcomes and promote their long-term health objectives.

# CHAPTER ONE

## The Biology Relating To Body Type Diet

Dr. Eric Berg's Body Type food is based on the idea that people can maximize their health and well-being by customizing their food and lifestyle to fit their unique body type. This customized approach is based on a thorough comprehension of the science underlying how hormones, metabolism, and heredity affect an individual's general health and body composition.

## Body Types And Genetics

Understanding the influence of genetics on a person's body type is a cornerstone of the Body Type Diet. Dr. Berg highlights the role that genetics plays in differences in body size, shape, and nutrient processing. People can better appreciate the uniqueness of their bodies and make educated decisions about their nutrition and lifestyle by being aware of and comprehending these hereditary impacts.

Genetic predispositions are used to classify several body kinds, including the liver, thyroid, ovary, and adrenal types. These categories are the basis for customizing dietary advice to target particular genetic inclinations.

For example, people with adrenal body types would benefit from an adrenal function-supporting diet, but others with thyroid body types might need a different dietary strategy to maximize their metabolism.

## Metabolic Processes And Body Structure

One of the main tenets of the Body Type Diet is metabolism, which is vital to understanding body composition. Dr. Berg stresses that creating a successful diet plan requires knowing one's metabolic rate. The diet offers specific suggestions to support a healthy metabolism and aid in weight management, accounting for individual differences in metabolic rates.

Different metabolic traits are linked to different body types. People who have a slow metabolism, for instance, can be categorized as liver types, whereas people who have a rapid metabolism might be classed as adrenal or thyroid body types. The Body Type Diet attempts to maximize energy levels, improve the body's ability to burn fat, and advance general health by customizing food choices to an individual's metabolic requirements.

## Hormones: Their Function

The Body Type Diet acknowledges the important role hormones play in regulating weight, mood, and energy levels, among other elements of health. Dr. Berg places a strong emphasis on the influence of hormones on body composition and metabolism, including insulin, cortisol, estrogen, and testosterone.

Through specific dietary therapies aimed at correcting hormonal imbalances, people may be able to enhance their health results.

Certain bodily forms are frequently linked to hormonal abnormalities. For instance, people with apple-shaped bodies may be more likely to be insulin resistant, whereas people with adrenal body types may be more susceptible to cortisol imbalances.

 The Body Type Diet provides dietary recommendations to maintain hormonal balance, enhance overall health, and treat particular issues associated with body types.

To sum up, the research underlying the Body Type Diet is complex and takes into account the complex interactions between hormones, metabolism, and heredity. Through comprehension and acceptance of these concepts, people can set out on a customized path to improved health by utilizing dietary and lifestyle decisions catered to their distinct body types.

# CHAPTER TWO

## Ectomorphs: The Type Of Lean Body

The body type diet theory is based on the notion that people may be divided into various body types, each of which has distinct traits and metabolic preferences. One such body type is the ectomorph, which is distinguished by a slim and lean physique.

Comprehending the unique characteristics of ectomorphs is crucial in customizing a diet and fitness regimen that corresponds with their requirements and objectives

.

# Eigenschaften Von Ectomorphen

Features including a quick metabolism, narrow shoulders, a slender build, and trouble gaining weight in both muscle and fat are common in ectomorphs. Even when they consume an excess of calories, they may find it difficult to gain weight because they frequently have a higher ratio of lean muscle mass to body weight. In addition to having smaller bones and joints generally, ectomorphs tend to seem slim overall.

Ectomorphs burn more calories than people with other body types when it comes to energy expenditure. This metabolic trait may affect how people react to specific diets and exercise regimens. To support their exercise and health goals, a customized strategy must take into account these innate features.

## Customizing Exercise And Nutrition For Ectomorphs

Ectomorphs have special needs when it comes to their food and exercise routines, so it's important to customize them accordingly. Ectomorphs frequently need to consume more calories to maintain muscle growth and to offset their rapid metabolism.

A macronutrient mix that is well-balanced and includes healthy fats, proteins, and carbs is essential for supplying the energy required for daily tasks as well as for the development of muscle.

For ectomorphs, protein consumption becomes especially important since it is essential for muscle growth and repair. It's crucial to include lean protein sources including fish, chicken, eggs, and plant-based proteins.

Incorporating foods high in nutrients and complex carbs also contributes to ensuring that there is a sufficient calorie surplus to support their fitness objectives.

When it comes to exercise, ectomorphs find that doing resistance and strength training activities together promotes muscular growth. Exercises like bench presses, deadlifts, and squats that use many muscular groups are examples of compound movements that can be very beneficial. To promote muscular hypertrophy, ectomorphs may need to train at a moderate to high intensity and concentrate on progressive overload.

## Examples Of Workouts And Meal Plans

Meal plans and exercise routines that are representative of ectomorphs might offer important insights into a practical strategy. The focus of meal plans should be on nutrient-dense foods that are distributed throughout the day in a balance of carbohydrates, proteins, and fats. A regular calorie intake can be achieved by eating smaller, more frequent meals and snacks.

To target different muscular areas, sample workouts for ectomorphs should combine isolation and complex exercises. A well-planned exercise program may incorporate aerobic, flexibility, and strength training exercises.

To properly allow muscles to mend and expand, it's critical to find a balance between effort and recovery.

Creating a body type diet that works for ectomorphs requires a thorough grasp of their distinct traits. In addition to fostering general health and well-being, adjusting food and exercise to this slim body type's unique requirements can help achieve ideal fitness outcomes.

# CHAPTER THREE

## Mesomorphs: The Type Of Athletic Body

A naturally larger percentage of lean muscle mass and a faster metabolism define mesomorphs' athletic and muscular build.

These people are good candidates for athletic endeavors because they tend to acquire and shed weight very easily. Mesomorphs are characterized by a traditional "V" shaped chest, shoulders, and hips.

It is essential to comprehend mesomorph characteristics to customize diet and exercise regimens that will maximize their physical potential.

# Features Of Metamorphs

Mesomorphs differ from other body types due to certain physical traits they possess.

They frequently have powerful, naturally athletic frames with well-defined muscles. Because of their generally faster metabolisms, mesomorphs find it simpler to burn calories and keep a healthy weight.

They might also find it relatively easy to gain muscular mass, which is beneficial for people who train for strength or participate in activities that call for endurance and power.

# Personalized Diet And Exercise Plans For Mesomorphs

Mesomorphs must customize their diet and exercise regimens to meet their unique needs to maintain optimal health and fitness.

A balanced diet with a variety of macronutrients and an emphasis on lean proteins to promote muscle growth is generally beneficial for mesomorphs.

It is frequently advised that they have a moderate amount of carbohydrates to fuel their active lifestyles and that they consume good fats for general well-being. Strength training and cardiovascular workouts work well together to assist mesomorphs in staying thin while maintaining their muscular mass.

## Useful Advice For Mesomorphs

Mesomorphs that apply these useful recommendations to their regular routines can maximize their athletic potential.

To keep their level of fitness well-rounded, it is recommended that they participate in a range of physical activities that incorporate both strength training and cardiovascular workouts.

Because mesomorphs may be more likely to experience weight changes, it is important to be cautious of calorie intake and portion control.

For optimum performance and general health, it's also crucial to prioritize recovery through enough rest and sleep and to stay hydrated.

Mesomorphs can create individualized plans for reaching their fitness objectives when they recognize and value their unique features.

 Mesomorphs can take advantage of their natural advantages and lead active, healthy lives by using a customized approach to training and diet.

# CHAPTER FOUR

## Endomorphs: The Type Of Curvy Body

Understanding individual variances in metabolism, physique, and responsiveness to different lifestyle circumstances is greatly aided by the concept of body types.

One of the three main body types is the endomorph, which is distinguished by its propensity to retain fat easily, its round or soft physique, and its generally curvaceous appearance.

Knowing what makes endomorphs different from other types of people will help you create diet and fitness regimens that will work best for them.

# Recognizing Endomorph Features

Endomorphs usually have physical characteristics that set them apart from other body types.

These characteristics include a propensity to gain weight more quickly, a slower metabolism, and a larger percentage of body fat, particularly in the stomach region.

Furthermore, endomorphs frequently have a curvier silhouette and a softer, more rounded body form. Comprehending and identifying these attributes is crucial in formulating focused approaches to cater to the distinct requirements of people with an endomorphic body type.

## Techniques For Endomorphs' Exercise And Nutrition

For people with an endomorphic body type, developing a customized diet and workout regimen is essential to reaching their fitness and health objectives. Endomorphs may benefit from a well-balanced diet that has an emphasis on portion management, nutrient-dense meals, and a modest intake of carbs due to their propensity to store fat quickly. Endomorphs can benefit from frequent aerobic activity, strength training, and high-intensity interval training (HIIT) to increase their metabolism and control their weight.

For endomorphs, it's critical to comprehend the significance of consistency in both nutrition and activity. Changing one's lifestyle in a way that encourages sustained adherence can aid with weight management and enhance general health.

 Making the approach unique to each person's tastes, nutritional demands, and level of fitness is essential to developing long-lasting habits that meet endomorphs' specific requirements.

## Ideas For Meals And Workout Programs

Meal preparation is essential to helping endomorphs achieve their fitness and health objectives. A nutrient-dense, well-balanced diet that includes a variety of lean proteins, whole grains, fruits, and vegetables can help with weight management and improve general health. Smaller, more frequent meals spread out throughout the day may also aid in controlling hunger and the metabolism.

Strength training, flexibility training, and aerobic activities should all be included in endomorph-specific fitness regimens. Yoga, weight training, jogging, and brisk walking are a few appropriate workout options.

Creating a fitness regimen that balances anaerobic and aerobic exercises can help you lose weight, gain muscle, and improve your general health.

Optimizing health and reaching fitness objectives requires an awareness of endomorph traits and the application of individualized diet and exercise plans. People with an endomorphic body type can start down the path to better health and long-lasting lifestyle modifications by adopting a comprehensive strategy that takes individual characteristics into account.

## Developing A Diet Plan For Your Body Type

Comprehending and executing a Body Type Diet plan entails customizing your exercise and dietary habits to your body type. This method recognizes that people differ in their physiological makeup, which affects how they react to certain diets and physical activities. This diet plan uses individualized ways to classify people into body types to maximize health and well-being.

## How To Create A Balanced Diet

Creating a comprehensive and balanced diet that fits your body type is an essential part of the Body Type Diet. The ectomorph, mesomorph, and endomorph body types each have unique dietary requirements. For example, ectomorphs might benefit from consuming more carbohydrates, mesomorphs might do well with a balanced macronutrient ratio, and endomorphs might need to watch their carbohydrate consumption carefully to maintain weight control. Achieving optimal health and fitness requires a focus on nutrient-dense diets and a suitable calorie balance.

Think about combining a range of entire foods, such as lean proteins, complex carbs, healthy fats, and an abundance of fruits and vegetables, into your diet to create a balanced one.

Adjust the ratios of these macronutrients to suit the needs of your particular body type. An individual's nutrition plan can be tailored to meet their specific physiological demands by taking into account factors like meal time, portion sizes, and the quality of food sources.

## Customizing Your Exercise Program

An effective Body Type Diet plan includes not only modifying your diet but also your exercise regimen to meet your body type and fitness objectives. Resistance training can help ectomorphs, who usually have a slim frame, gain muscular mass. Mesomorphs, who have more of an athletic and muscular build, should concentrate on a well-rounded fitness regimen that incorporates both cardiovascular and strength training. Weight management for endomorphs, who tend to accumulate more body fat, may benefit from a combination of resistance training and aerobic activity.

Knowing your body type will help you modify your exercise program to get the most out of it and improve your general health. A sustained fitness regimen can be aided by selecting things you enjoy doing, as consistency is crucial. Whether you work with weights, aerobics, yoga, or a mix of activities, customizing your fitness routine to your body type will help you reach your fitness goals.

## Having Reasonable Objectives

Setting attainable goals that fit your particular body type and way of life is a crucial component of the Body Type Diet plan. This method encourages people to set tailored goals based on their unique body type traits, as opposed to following general criteria.

A realistic objective takes into consideration your body type, current level of fitness, and how quickly your body adjusts to changes in diet and exercise.

Take into account both immediate and long-term goals when establishing goals. While long-term objectives offer a more comprehensive view of your journey toward health and fitness, short-term goals can help you stay motivated and monitor your progress.

Pay attention to how your body reacts to changes in your diet and exercise routine, and adjust as necessary. Savor minor triumphs during the journey, acknowledging that advancements could differ depending on personal elements. You can improve your chances of long-term success in attaining and sustaining a healthy lifestyle with the Body Type Diet by setting individualized, attainable goals.

# CHAPTER FIVE

## Extomorphetic Recipe Books:

Ectomorphs are people with a slim and lean build who frequently have a quick metabolism and have trouble acquiring weight.

Foods high in calories and nutrients that promote muscular building should be the main emphasis of their diet. Recipes that are suitable for ectomorphs have a strong emphasis on a ratio of protein to carbs and healthy fats.

Lean proteins like chicken or fish, complex carbs like sweet potatoes or quinoa, and generous portions of veggies to supply vital vitamins and minerals can all be found in meals. These recipes are designed to support muscle growth and assist ectomorphs in satisfying their calorie needs.

## Approved Meals For Mesomorphs:

Mesomorphs are people that naturally have an athletic build, with defined muscles and a fast metabolism. A balanced diet with a moderate distribution of macronutrients seems to work well for the mesomorph body type. Meals that are suitable for mesomorphs emphasize lean proteins to help with muscle building and maintenance, complex carbohydrates to provide long-lasting energy, and healthy fats for general well-being. With a balanced and nourishing diet, these dishes will help the mesomorph maintain their shape and improve their athletic performance.

## Dishes Particular To Endomorphs:

Endomorphs tend to be softer, rounder-built, and to store more fat on their bodies. For endomorphs, controlling weight and maximizing metabolism are crucial factors. Dishes tailored to endomorphs are made to increase fullness, curb cravings, and aid in weight loss.

Lean proteins to help maintain muscle mass, high-fiber carbs to moderate blood sugar levels, and an emphasis on portion control are common ingredients in these dishes. These recipes use nutrient-dense ingredients to assist endomorphs in reaching and maintaining a healthy weight while taking into account their unique metabolic traits.

The Body Type Diet provides a customized approach to eating by acknowledging the differences in people's bodies and metabolisms. The ectomorph, mesomorph, and endomorph recipes are tailored to the specific requirements of each body type to promote total well-being, support fitness objectives, and maximize health.

Adopting a diet that is in line with one's body type enables people to make decisions that support their unique fitness and health goals.

# CHAPTER SIX

## Overcoming Implications And Difficulties

When pursuing the Body Type Diet, individuals may run into obstacles and roadblocks on their path to reaching their fitness and health objectives. These challenges must be overcome to make consistent progress and follow the recommended dietary recommendations.

## Handling Stagnations

It is not unusual to experience plateaus in either muscle building or weight loss; the Body Type Diet provides ways to overcome them. These can involve altering the workout regimen, tweaking the ratios of macronutrients, or implementing periodic adjustments to overcome plateaus and encourage continuous improvement.

## Typical Problems And Their Fixes

The Body Type Diet may provide several obstacles during implementation, including controlling appetites or following particular food requirements. Creating a customized food plan, getting advice from nutritionists, and adjusting the diet to suit each person's preferences are typical remedies.

## Remaining Inspired

For any diet plan to be successful over the long run, motivation must be maintained. The Body Type Diet acknowledges the role that psychological variables have in reaching health objectives.

Setting attainable goals, acknowledging accomplishments, and maintaining an optimistic outlook are some techniques for maintaining motivation to adhere to dietary recommendations.

# CHAPTER SEVEN

## Including The Body-Type Diet In Your Daily Living

According to Dr. Abravanel's Body Type Diet, a person's body type might influence their metabolic rate and, in turn, the diet that is best for them.

Knowing your body type—pituitary, gonadal, adrenal, or thyroid—is essential to adjusting your diet to promote general health.

A comprehensive strategy that takes into account all facets of daily life is necessary to successfully incorporate the Body Type Diet into your way of life.

## Getting Together And Dining Out

Following a certain diet can be difficult when attending social events and eating out. On the other hand, handling these circumstances gets easier while following the Body Type Diet.

For instance, it may be advantageous for those with adrenal body types to eat meals high in vegetables and lean proteins and low in carbs. Similar to this, people with thyroid body types might concentrate on a mixture of carbohydrates, fats, and proteins that is well-balanced. Making educated decisions at social gatherings guarantees that your food selections complement your body type without sacrificing the fun of dining out and interacting with others.

## Traveling While Keeping Your Diet In Check

Traveling frequently throws routines off, which makes following a diet plan difficult. The Body Type Diet recognizes this and offers people on-the-go flexibility.

Knowing your body type helps you choose wisely from the variety of food options available, whether you're traveling for work or pleasure. Maintaining your nutritional objectives when traveling can be facilitated by bringing along wholesome foods that suit your body type and doing some prior study on the local cuisine. You may balance exploration with nutrition by implementing the Body Type Diet's tenets into your vacation itinerary.

## Juggling Career And Health

Keeping up a healthy lifestyle while handling job obligations is a typical problem. Your professional life can be enhanced by the customized approach to nutrition provided by The Body Type Diet. For example, to maintain energy levels during the workday, people with pituitary body types may benefit from a diet emphasizing a balance of proteins, lipids, and carbs. You can further support your overall health goals by including activity and brief breaks for mindful eating in your daily routine. The Body

Type Diet can be smoothly incorporated into your professional life if you strike a balance between your work obligations and body type-based health-conscious decisions.

Incorporating the Body Type Diet into your lifestyle entails modifying its tenets for a variety of situations in everyday life. Understanding your body type enables you to make smart food decisions that promote your general well-being, whether you're socializing, traveling, or juggling work. You can successfully combine the demands of an active lifestyle with health-conscious living by implementing the Body Type Diet into your daily routine.

## The Body-Mind Relationship

The idea of the mind-body connection highlights the complex interrelationship between physical and mental health. It suggests that a person's physical and mental well-being are strongly correlated. Understanding this relationship becomes essential for attaining overall health and well-being in the context of the body type diet. Our general state of health is significantly shaped by the interaction of psychological variables and physiological processes.

## Physical Types And Emotional Eating

Emotional eating is a phenomenon in which people eat to deal with their emotions rather than because they are physically hungry. The body type diet acknowledges the connection between certain body types and emotional eating. Different body types may become involved in harmful eating behaviors due to specific emotional triggers.

It becomes crucial to recognize and comprehend these triggers to modify dietary recommendations to meet not only bodily but also emotional needs.

## Conscious Eating Techniques

Being completely present and paying close attention when ingesting food is the foundation of the mindful eating practice. Contemplative eating extends beyond calorie tracking and restrictive meal plans in the framework of the body-type diet. It promotes people to develop a keen awareness of their eating preferences, routines, and the feelings that come with eating.

A more sustainable and well-rounded lifestyle can be fostered by helping people cultivate a better relationship with food through the integration of mindfulness into the dietary approach.

## Stress Reduction Methods

A key component of the body type diet is stress management, which recognizes the significant negative effects of stress on mental and physical health.

Different body types respond to stress differently in the body, which affects things like hormone balance and metabolism. To lessen the damaging effects of stress on the body, the diet includes stress management practices. This could involve techniques like deep breathing exercises, meditation, and other body-type-specific stress-reduction techniques.

To sum up, the body type diet is based on the mind-body link, which acknowledges the complex relationship between mental and physical health.

Through the application of stress management strategies, mindful eating practices, and an understanding of body types, people can tackle emotional eating and take a comprehensive approach to better health and vitality.

# CHAPTER EIGHT

## Fitness Outside Of Diet

A vital component of overall health that goes beyond food choices is fitness. Maintaining optimal health requires not just a good and well-balanced diet, but also a variety of exercise regimens. The Body Type Diet is a comprehensive approach that highlights the importance of customizing exercise regimens for each particular body type.

### Including A Range Of Exercise Techniques

Realizing that various body types react to exercise in different ways is one of the fundamental tenets of the Body Type Diet. Knowing one's body type might help in creating a fitness regimen that fits specific requirements and objectives. A holistic approach to fitness is ensured by the combination of multiple exercise modalities, including aerobic workouts, strength training, and flexibility exercises.

Running, cycling, and swimming are examples of cardiovascular exercises that are crucial for strengthening the heart and burning calories. On the other hand, the goals of strength training are to increase metabolism and muscle mass. Stretching and yoga are examples of flexibility activities that improve general mobility and reduce the risk of injury. People can address different parts of fitness and meet the unique needs of their body type by varying the types of workouts they do.

Creating a Long-Term Exercise Program

The Body Type Diet places a strong emphasis on developing a sustainable fitness regimen. The goal is to create long-lasting habits rather than committing to severe exercise routines or passing on transitory trends. To produce long-lasting effects and advance general well-being, sustainability is essential.

Individual fitness levels, schedule constraints, and personal preferences are all taken into account in a sustainable fitness regimen. To avoid burnout and injuries, it promotes a steady increase in both time and intensity. Customizing the regimen to meet personal demands increases the likelihood of adherence, which promotes long-term success in upholding an active and healthy lifestyle.

## The Advantages Of Yoga For Various Body Types

Yoga is an important part of the Body Type Diet because of its many forms and flexibility.

In addition to improving bodily health, this age-old practice also tends to mental and emotional health. Yoga is beneficial for all body types, so it's a great complement to any exercise regimen.

Those with an ectomorphic body type—which is characterized by a slim build—may find that yoga helps them relax and tone their muscles. Mesomorphic body types—typified by a more muscular build—can profit from the flexibility and balancing elements of yoga. Yoga may help endomorphic people, who have a propensity to retain fat, control their weight, and reduce stress.

The Body Type nutrition highlights the significance of customizing exercise regimens to specific body types and highlights that fitness transcends nutrition. Through the integration of several exercise modalities, the development of enduring fitness regimens, and the acknowledgment of the advantages of yoga, individuals can attain a comprehensive approach to health and wellness.

# Conclusion

In conclusion, by classifying people into distinct body types, the Body Type Diet provides a customized approach to eating. The dietary suggestions are customized to address the emotional, hormonal, and metabolic traits specific to each type. Despite the growing popularity of the Body Type Diet, it is important to approach any diet critically and seek the guidance of healthcare specialists for specific recommendations.

Several important ideas come to light as the Body Type Diet is examined. First and foremost, there is the notion that a person's hormones, metabolism, and emotional inclinations are all influenced by their body form. Comprehending these variables is essential to customizing a diet that meets personal requirements. Each of the four dietary types—thyroid, adrenal, ovarian, and liver—has unique dietary guidelines to maximize health.

Due to their quick metabolism, people with Thyroid Types benefit from diets high in iodine and selenium, which promote thyroid function.

Adrenal Types, who have a slower metabolism and are more sensitive to stress, concentrate on controlling cortisol levels by choosing certain foods and eating at certain times. For those with ovarian types who struggle with hormonal imbalances, cruciferous vegetables, and high-fiber foods are key components of a diet that regulates estrogen levels. Liver types that are linked to a slow metabolism and weight accumulation in the abdomen concentrate on enhancing liver function by eating foods that detoxify the liver.

## Anticipating A Healthier Future

When people contemplate implementing the Body Type Diet or any other customized nutrition strategy, it's critical to have a balanced future-focused outlook. Although the idea of customizing meals to fit specific traits is appealing, it's important to remember that nutrition is a complicated topic and that people react differently to different foods. To live a healthy future, one must take into account not only their body type but also a holistic approach to well-being that includes consistent exercise, enough hydration, and mindful eating practices generally. A sustained and individualized approach to nutrition and well-being as one travels the path to better health requires knowledge, professional consultation, and bodily awareness.

www.ingramcontent.com/pod-product-compliance
Lightning Source LLC
Chambersburg PA
CBHW060802260726

48660CB00002B/731